SELF-CARE STRATEGIES FOR 24/7 MOMS

SIMPLE SOLUTIONS TO RESET, RELAX, AND RECHARGE

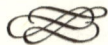

REESE FRAZIER

TRILLIUM SAGE
PUBLISHING

ISBN 978-1-958118-02-3/Ebook ISBN 978-1-958118-01-6

Trillium Sage Publishing | www.trilliumsage.com

3943 Irvine Blvd #138, Irvine, CA 92602, USA

To all the exhausted mamas out there...

You got this!

CONTENTS

INTRODUCTION

Wow, that mom looks tired.

And then it hit me. *I* was *that* mom years ago! I was that mom who woke up even before the sun rose, getting ready to prepare *everything* for the family. I was that mom who had her hair tied up in a messy bun all the time - walking with a newborn tucked close to her chest in a sling, cruising through the neighborhood pushing a stroller with a two-year-old inside and a four-year-old next to her, his hand holding onto her shirt. There were days when I would release a huge sigh of relief whenever those three little monkeys went to bed extra early - even if it was only 15 minutes earlier than their usual bedtime.

But that is history. My three sons are now in their stinky teenage years - meaning they can do things by themselves. I no longer sit by the bathtub, waiting for them to finish playing with their squirt guns or trying to figure out how to feed them medicine when they run a fever. I rarely feel physically exhausted since they've become teens, but another problem arises. I'm now mentally and emotionally tired.

Looking at myself in the mirror, the messy bun is gone, but so is the glow in my face. Trust me when I say this - a worn-out mind is way worse than an exhausted body. It strips away everything in you. So, when I catch myself in this state, I know it's time - time to do what I must do to recharge. As my schedule allows, I mentally run through a myriad of options available to reset *myself*. I'm confident that I'll be in a much better state after doing just a little something *for me*. Whether it be sitting quietly with a strong cup of coffee, taking the dog out for a long walk, or getting away for the weekend with my best friend (usually involving a bit of wine, of course) - I will surely return well-rested and ready to get back to mom-ing.

The urge to fully reboot myself grew even more vital when I was widowed with three young sons. At the age of 41, I lost my parenting co-pilot, and I was left with zero choices but to do this alone. I wasn't just a single parent now; I was an *only* parent. I would be lying if I said that I was not overwhelmed by the daily grind of raising my boys, so the only thing that could save me from this never-ending exhaustion was to make self-care one of my top priorities. After I made that conscious decision, I'm thrilled to say that I finally achieved the balance between rest and responsibility.

You might be familiar with an old adage - *you can't pour from an empty cup.* Those words hit me like a ton of bricks, and I can vouch for their accuracy. Moms, it must start with *you.* Always. You can never take care of others if you don't care for *yourself* first, just like those pre-flight instructions. *Passengers, please wear your oxygen mask before helping others.* As moms, we are a massive part of the family, and everyone depends on us, so we need to be in top form all the time.

Once you have taken this baby step to make yourself a priority, part of the heavy load on your shoulders will be gone. You'll slowly regain your glow and realize that you actually have ample space to breathe. This can be achieved *without* neglecting your role as a parent – as you'll soon see.

We'll first start by diving deeper into the actual benefit of self-care and how it can bring out the best version of you that you might not even know exists! So, first things first - flip the page and continue reading as I walk you through this journey of finding that perfect balance between rest and responsibility, step by step.

ONE

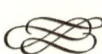

THE IMPORTANCE OF SELF-CARE

Moms, before we begin, let's say this together: Self-care is not merely a suggestion for a healthy family. It is a *necessity!* Keep on repeating this mantra to yourself over and over again.

Now, let's take a trip down memory lane when you were pregnant with your first child, and self-care was the ultimate priority in your life. I'm a hundred percent sure that you took every necessary precaution to take care of yourself for your baby's well-being. You probably took your prenatal vitamins, drank a ridiculous amount of water every day, met with your doctors regularly, and resisted alcohol and sushi (the latter proved to be most challenging for me). Just like how you took complete care of your well-being for the sake of your unborn child back then, self-care is still as important even after you've given birth. Not a thing has changed since then - you still *need* to take good care of yourself for your child's well-being. The only difference is that your child is no longer in your womb and your feet aren't swollen all the time.

Of course, I won't deny that we moms always want the best for our families. Yet that does not mean that we can't take a break at all. Just imagine this – you take a short break on the weekend by going out to dinner with your best friend, returning home with a less stressed-out mind. You can give more to your children when you have a clear mind, and more than likely, you'll have more patience when they're up to their antics.

You won't believe the dozens of benefits that you can gain just by implementing self-care into your life. Being deliberate and investing the time and energy to care for yourself will not only reward you with a clear mind, but it will also grant you multiple long-term advantages such as:

- reduced anxiety and depression
- relief from stress
- a positive mindset
- a boost to your self-esteem
- increased productivity
- staying healthy

These benefits of self-care extend way beyond yourself. Your family will greatly benefit from you taking some time off to care for yourself as well. When I was too overwhelmed, I could blow a fuse at the snap of a finger. When I lost my temper because of tiny, trivial matters, I realized that I was far from the mom I wanted to be for my sons. Who wants a snappy, short-tempered mom who keeps nagging at everyone? My kids sure didn't! Goodness, I wouldn't want that either! So, long story short, a well-cared for mom will definitely make a happier home for everyone.

Another significant positive impact of taking care of yourself is that it will help you avoid burnout. Moms are notorious for sacrificing themselves for the good of the family, and I don't know any mom who is not at risk of burning out. Even though you believe that it is your responsibility to give 110% to your family, believe me, as time passes, you'll somewhat feel a tinge of depression slowly consuming you. You might not notice this right away, but it will happen if you overwork and don't prioritize yourself.

Over time, burnout will eventually manifest as physical symptoms that are difficult for you to ignore. If you are feeling any of the symptoms below, it might indicate that you are beginning to experience burnout and need some self-care immediately.

- Changes in sleeping or eating habits
- More frequent headaches, dizziness, or upset stomach
- Feeling unsafe, unhappy, guilty, anxious, or lonely
- Having difficulty concentrating
- Feeling withdrawn and being easily irritated
- Having multiple crying bouts or angry outbursts

These symptoms carry a domino effect. Once you experience an irregular sleeping schedule, you'll wake up the following day already feeling on edge. These uncomfortable feelings will lead you to the next stage - stressed out, unhappy, anxious, and everything in between. Worst case scenario - if you continue to ignore these red flags, you'll finally feel withdrawn and might end the day with multiple outbursts of anger and tears. The last thing you want to do is to lash out in anger at the kids and regret it a second later.

I've experienced burnout firsthand. I suppose I could check off each of the symptoms above when my eldest son was still in elementary school, and his younger brothers were in preschool. During that time, I was aware that I was not in my best form, but at the same time, I had no clue why I felt that way - in my cluttered mind, nothing was wrong. My sons were doing great. The whole house was squeaky clean; everything was in order. So, I consulted a medical professional. After a few minutes of scanning through my symptoms, he diagnosed me with exhaustion. There I was, listening to my doctor explain what I was experiencing and felt rather surprised thinking that only celebrities suffered from exhaustion!

The doctor then wrote me a note and ordered me to rest for two solid weeks. *How could a mom take it easy and do nothing for two weeks straight with so many chores on deck?* But the doctor gave me a stern look, and I could only obey for the sake of my health. While I was on medical leave, I relied on my husband and my parents to assist me with family duties, and I felt even more guilty because it was as if I had caused an inconvenience to them. So, lesson learned - I can't get myself in this situation again. I better slow down my pace and begin taking better care of myself.

But, of course, you can't make drastic changes and expect to see results immediately. You need to take one step at a time, and eventually, you'll start to feel the difference. So, let's move on to the next chapter and start changing our routine!

TWO

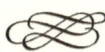

BASIC FOUNDATIONAL HABITS

When I ask moms out there why they do not apply self-care in their routine, the answers that I gathered are mostly the same. Some say that it's almost impossible to get free time away from their kids, let alone book an appointment for a manicure at the nail salon. Some say that they don't have enough wiggle room in their budget for a short weekend getaway with friends or a night out. Most people often mistake self-care with self-indulgence. So, to dispel those negative stereotypes, I'm here to inform you that self-care does not have to be about pampering yourself with a luxurious facial or treating yourself to expensive gourmet dishes! You can be sitting in the living room in your favorite pajamas while bingeing Netflix or spending fifteen minutes exercising in your backyard while the children are at school and still call it self-care.

Don't get me wrong, spending a couple of hours at the salon or the spa are great ideas too, but if you don't have the time for that or if you can't fit that into your financial situation, there are many more ways for you to apply self-care in your life. For starters, you can establish simple healthy habits to ensure you don't get overwhelmed by your daily tasks. The key here is not to overcomplicate self-care. These habits can work wonders and at least clear your mind, giving you a better chance for success.

One of the best ways to introduce self-care into your life is by creating a consistent morning routine. This step will keep your day well-organized and contribute to your peace of mind. Handling housework and dealing with your kids will be so much easier and fun if you're not feeling pressured and stressed all the time.

In summary, this is my morning routine:

- wake up at least 30 minutes before the family
- spend five minutes of quiet time
- make the bed
- take a quick shower
- get dressed
- drink a glass of water with lemon

I prefer getting up at least half an hour before the rest of the family. Doing so prevents me from rushing through my packed schedule, and I can have some quiet time to go through my daily chores and routines. These precious minutes before I 'clock into' work as a stay-at-home mom are one of my favorite parts of the day. I can have the time to myself and enjoy a warm, relaxing shower without my kids banging on the door asking if I've seen their misplaced items. After the shower, I can even spend a couple of minutes in front of my dresser, planning which shirt goes with which pants, and peacefully brew a hot cup of coffee to kick-start the long day.

Of course, getting out of bed super early in the morning can be a challenge even for us moms who have been doing it for years. As soon as you open your eyes, thinking about all the work that needs to be done for the day can cause you to stare blankly into space and create unnecessary stress in your mind. So, instead of focusing on the tasks, spend the first five minutes praying, meditating, or focusing on gratitude. The goal here is to take advantage of the stillness of the house and empty your mind. When I first started doing this, I managed to start the day with a sense of calm.

To certain people (like yours truly), making the bed can be therapeutic. Doing this somehow gives a sense that I've accomplished the first task of the day, and it encourages me to complete the next ones. Another thing that you should pay attention to before you start doing anything else is the way you dress. This might surprise you, but believe it or not, our appearance and how we dress can impact our productivity. You don't have to choose something fancy, but try to wear something presentable, neat, and comfortable at the very least. How we dress is heavily linked to us feeling good about ourselves, so seeing yourself in decent clothes will significantly motivate you to complete your tasks throughout the day.

Moms are real-life superheroes as we can do things simultaneously. At one time, you can be in the kitchen, juggling between preparing breakfast and feeding your toddler while answering your four-year-old's endless questions. So, how can you stay energized for the rest of the day, you ask? Simple - hydration is the key! Before you jump into any chores on your list, get to the kitchen, and pour yourself a glass of water. Your body does not consume water while you're sleeping, and seven to eight hours is a long period of time to go without any water. So, drinking a glass in the morning can help you rehydrate your body and boost your brain efficiency. I recommend adding a slice of lemon, too, as it can improve your digestion.

After you check off a few items from your list, it's time to take a short break and refresh your mind. One of the best ways to do this is to get out of the house for some fresh air. There's no need to drive somewhere to do this; instead, you can just hang around your backyard, balcony, or porch. Take in a few deep breaths, look at the calming blue color of the skies and relax for a bit. It'll be even better if you do some simple exercises. Fun fact - our brains produce a hormone called serotonin when we exercise, which is responsible for making us feel happy. Not only will you have more energy, but you'll also be in a better mood and feel more optimistic after a short workout.

In addition to getting yourself used to a simple workout routine every morning, it's also a good idea to include healthy meals in your day. As we are all aware, a well-balanced diet can significantly impact both our physical and mental health. According to studies, too much consumption of unhealthy food can lead to stress and depression (Sutter Health, n.d.). Try your best to avoid processed food no matter how busy you are and replace it with food rich in nutrients. In my case, salmon is my go-to. There are many ways to prepare salmon – I prefer mine either raw as sushi or roasted with some greens on the side – both taste amazing! According to Hjalmars-dottir (2018), salmon is rich in omega-3 fatty acids, reducing your risks of getting heart disease and helping you fight depression and anxiety. Don't forget, water too is part of a healthy diet. So, try to at least drink 80 ounces of water every day.

Now that we got some of the basics down with what we do as part of our daily morning routine, let's next consider what we can do to care for ourselves for the rest of the day.

It's okay to say 'no.' There's a reason why that word exists, and it is not rude or selfish to use it!

This is your second mantra. Say it to yourself repeatedly. Don't forget, it's perfectly fine to say 'no' sometimes. Don't overcommit yourself, especially when you have a ton of chores that day. I understand that declining a request can make you feel guilty because I once felt that same exact way. I just felt so guilty to let the word 'no' escape from my lips. Yet the truth is, just like every other person in this world, you have your priorities. Overcommitting and saying 'yes' to everything will only overwhelm you and lead to stress. Don't worry about other people's perceptions of you. Saying 'no' shows that you know your priority and value. Creating this boundary will save you in the long run.

Staying organized can also help you maintain a healthy mind. I'm not going to lie, but even thinking about what to cook for breakfast, lunch, and dinner for the next day can stress me out sometimes. To overcome this, I began meal planning for the week ahead. You can jot it down in your planner or just on a piece of paper and put it on your refrigerator - anything that works for you. By doing this, you no longer have to worry every single night about what dish you will be preparing the next day. Another tip for staying organized is to clean up your house before heading to bed. Put everything back in its place and make sure the whole space is tidy so that you won't wake up the following day and be greeted with messy surroundings. Trust me, laying eyes on an unkempt area early in the morning can quickly get my day off on the wrong foot!

When it comes to sleeping, try your best to have a consistent bedtime routine. It's highly recommended to get at least get seven hours of sleep every night. It might sound tempting to stay up after everyone has gone to bed as the whole house will become cozy and quiet, but you'll suffer the next day. You won't be well-rested if you stay up late and that's the last thing you want. If you can't find yourself sleeping due to an occupied mind, I'd suggest you do a 'brain dump.' This method only requires a piece of paper and a pen. Jot down everything that's occupying your mind and let it all out - you'll feel better, I promise! Take a few minutes to meditate and think of your success for the day, even if the achievement is something silly. One more thing that I never fail to do before calling it a day is spending some time reading. In my case, I prefer reading from a physical book compared to phones and tablets, as the light from devices makes it harder for me to hit the hay.

When I was overwhelmed and stressed out back then, my therapist strongly suggested that I be more deliberate to make time to clear my mind. Ideally, at least an hour of rest is needed every day. About two to three hours of self-care should be factored into your schedule every week and, if possible, a weekend off occasionally. You'll be one step closer to achieving a balance between rest and responsibility if you practice these essential habits. Once you've laid the proper foundation with these habits, we can move on to the next chapter to discuss self-care ideas that should be done on a daily basis.

THREE

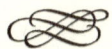

DAY TO DAY

Overwhelmed, stressed, and burned out – these are three of the main nemeses in a mother's life. Once you've encountered all three of them, you'll realize that you're now standing on your tippy toes underwater, just a few inches away from being completely drowned. At this time, the only hand that can reach out to save you from sinking is *yours*. I suppose you might have read about self-care before, and deep down, you acknowledge that it is necessary. Recognizing its importance is one thing, but implementing it into your daily life is a whole different matter.

Moms, including myself, tend to feel guilty when we take some time off - even if it's just a short fifteen minutes. We have this mindset that we are a foundation or the central pillar of the family and that if we stop working just for a short amount of time, everything will come crashing down. Half of it is true, we are the main foundation holding the family together, but mothers are human beings, too. We need a few moments to ourselves to recharge and return with a clearer mind. It doesn't matter whether you're a stay-at-home mom or a working-outside-of-the-home mom; you are your family's sunshine, the primary source of nourishment and comfort. You can't give them a mother's gentle touch if you don't take care of yourself first. So remember, your decision to start applying self-care is not only for yourself but also for your precious family.

Taking care of your mental state is far different from making sure you're physically healthy. Self-care is not just about eating healthy meals. Nor is it just about treating yourself to a high-end designer purse. Self-care is about doing a particular activity that brings joy to you and acts as a barrier keeping you from falling into a pool of stress. Remember that just because this one activity *seems* suitable for you does not make it self-care. You might have read or heard that going for a jog early in the morning can contribute to a healthy mind, but if you hate running, then it's not self-care for you! So, what else can you do daily that can act as your very own self-care routine?

Unleash your Creativity

If getting creative can make your day, then spending some time painting might work for you. Grab a canvas or even just a piece of paper, a couple of paintbrushes, and some paint. I prefer to create my masterpieces using acrylic paint as it dries quickly. You can do this while your kids are at school or when your little toddlers are asleep. Sit outside with an ice-cold glass of fresh lemonade, paint a serene landscape that you imagine in your mind, or even better, color a mandala. There are surprisingly many benefits of coloring a mandala. Studies suggest that not only can mandalas increase your creativity, but this can also act as a form of meditation as you allow your muscles to relax and help you reduce stress and anxiety (Steiss, n.d.).

I've found keeping a journal to be incredibly therapeutic. You can pour your thoughts into a journal to which only *you* have access. It's not necessary to churn out a 500-word essay every day; you can simply write down your feelings or any exciting events that you experienced that day, however minor. Bullet journals have been increasingly popular in recent years. If I had nothing to write, I'd settle down for a few minutes and list ten things that make me happy. This method can distract you from feeling pressured by your tasks and reset your mind again, making you feel more motivated to finish the remaining chores. I also keep three simple journals for my kids on my bedside table, and I try to write a short blurb about them at least once a week. I'll reread them once I've done a few pages, and it never fails to put a smile on my face. You can also write a letter to your loved ones and send it via snail mail. Since the world has gone digital with most communication, sending and receiving letters the traditional way is quite rare these days. I can assure you that getting a stamped envelope with your name and address is definitely more exciting than getting a notification on your phone!

Make Use of Social Media Platforms

Take advantage of social media - you can create an Instagram account to post pictures of things that bring you happiness, such as beautiful vistas, food that you've creatively plated, videos of your kids doing silly things, or even photos of your dog. It's your account, so your rules! If you must do small chores like the laundry or even slicing garlic for your aglio e olio, you can take away the dreariness of a mundane chore by listening to a podcast or to music. Create a music playlist filled with songs that remind you of happy times (I love my '80s playlist!) and listen to them while working - it'll be more fun and can improve your mood, especially while you're cleaning.

Parallel Reading

For moms who prefer reading as a way to relax, instead of reading a book alone, try reading a book in parallel with a friend. This way, you can connect with them and spend quality time discussing each other's takeaways.

GET OUT OF THE HOUSE FOR A LITTLE WHILE

Don't go straight home if you drive your little munchkins to school. Take a short drive nearby to get some fresh air. For some people (count me in), driving can act as an escape where you get a chance to be alone and clear your mind. Put on your favorite playlist and enjoy the ride. Sometimes, all you might need is a change of scenery to help you with your stressful moments. Getting outside and spending some time under the sun will not only supply your daily dose of Vitamin D, but it can also invigorate you. If you have a furry family member, take the dog for a walk. My dog gets crazy excited as soon as he sees his leash! Watching him jump around and wag his tail absolutely brightens my day.

CREATE A PERSONAL SPA

If you don't have time to go to the spa for a couple of hours relaxing and lying about, turn the house into your own private little spa. Diffuse calming essential oils to create a sense of peace. Try using spearmint or bergamot, which are known to soothe your emotions and reduce tension (McDermott, 2019). You can also opt for lavender, the most common aromatherapy scent packed with many benefits. Take ten minutes to meditate while listening to soothing sounds. After that, get a bubble bath ready and light the bathroom with a candle or two. Get in the tub, close your eyes, slowly breathe in and out and enjoy the quiet moment. Put on a face mask and enjoy the serenity of the moment. All of this can easily be done in less than an hour.

Get Something for Yourself While Grocery Shopping

One of my favorite parts of being a mom is that I get to go grocery shopping. There are two reasons for that: Grocery shopping makes me feel like I'm a legit adult and I have a responsibility. So, there's a sense of pride coming in when I've fulfilled this. Another reason is that I allocate some of my personal budget to purchasing things *I* want. For me, most of the time, it's a bottle of wine, a pint of ice cream, or occasionally, a bouquet of flowers. So, moms, try to set aside a budget to get what *you* want as well, not only the essential things for the household. Does a colorful bouquet of tulips make you happy? Then get one for yourself; no one can say 'no' to you. Are you craving a bar of decadent dark chocolate? Push your cart to the candy aisle and grab one. Never forget to ask what *you* want, too!

Get an Hour of Alone Time

When is the right time to enjoy those favorite items you bought from the store? The entire house is yours after you tuck the kids into bed and kiss them goodnight.

Ah... it's my favorite time of the day - happy hour! Pour a glass of the wine you've recently bought, bring your chocolate bar or bowl of ice cream to the couch, and cozy up. Press the Netflix button on the remote and watch an episode of your favorite show while enjoying those little treats. Be mindful, however, of your couch time and don't succumb to binge-watching an entire season - you need to get enough *zzzs* if you want to have a great day tomorrow.

While it is essential to take a short break from time to time, try to be realistic with your schedule. Don't fit these activities into your list because you've read it. Some people don't get true serenity by lighting aromatic candles or reading a book. Stay true to yourself - if taking a quiet drive can calm your mind, then include it in your self-care routine. If you're not a fan of writing, don't force yourself to keep a journal. Would taking a power nap can help you feel refreshed? Then do it. After all, self-care is about doing something that you are passionate about so that it can function as an escape from getting sucked into the quicksand.

Here are additional ideas you might consider incorporating into your daily schedule:

- plan a simple surprise for the kids, such as an after-school ice cream run, breakfast for dinner, or anything out of the ordinary

- create a vision board full of magazine clippings of things that make you smile
- write a sweet note to your children or spouse and place it somewhere to be found later
- take a few short minutes to brainstorm or daydream about where you want to go and what you want to do on your future getaway
- open up the AirBnb app and save your favorite homes for a future vacation
- list things that are stressing you out on a piece of paper, crumple it up, and throw it away
- print out a recent favorite photo and frame it up
- create a wish list on Amazon and dump everything that caught your attention in it (I love digital window shopping!)
- take a quick cold shower to refresh yourself
- blast a song and take five minutes to dance in the living room
- drop everything you're doing and do some stretching

I hope this short list will spark some ideas about what you can do to break up your daily routine. Let's see what we can do weekly in the next chapter.

FOUR

ONCE A WEEK

Let's hop in the time machine and set the date back to when you were in your early twenties, single, and actively traveling from one city to the next on weekends. Didn't it feel great? You've been working hard all week long, and to reward yourself, you decide to spend the entire weekend relaxing at home without laying a single finger on your laptop to check your emails. Either that or you dial up your close friends and go out for an impromptu girls' trip with an itinerary full of wine tasting and a spa day. You had a blast and returned home with a lighter mind, ready to get back to work the next day. Now, let's get back to the present time and ask yourself - why did I stop doing those things? Why did I stop rewarding myself after getting through a stressful week? Is it because I don't deserve that anymore since I'm now a mom? Of course not!

When you were younger, you worked 9 to 5 to 'take care' of your company or business. When you're a mother, you're working to take care of your family, and there are no standard business hours for parenting! You're there for your loved ones 24/7. You can't just ignore your five-year-old crying in the middle of the night because of a nightmare like how you occasionally miss your email notifications. You carry different roles at home, from a chef to a teacher to a chauffeur, and if you have kids like mine, at times, a referee. You have loads of tasks on your plate, and you accomplish everything by the end of each day. So why shouldn't you reward yourself at the end of the week?

Time constraints might be an issue. I had problems with time management myself. Back then, I always failed to find enough time to do the things that I enjoyed - I couldn't even find 20 minutes to go out and walk the dog. But I learned one thing that changed everything. The secret to finding more time is to *prioritize!* You can't just sit around and wait for the extra time to land on your lap. Plus, there is no spare time - 24 hours a day is all you've got, and that's that. So, it's up to you to set your priorities and use the time you that you *do* have. There's an hour left before the kids return from school, and you've completed all your chores? Use that time to do something you like instead of *searching* for more tasks to complete.

So, how do you plan a weekly activity to ensure you're always in a good mental state? Of course, unlike when you had no children, you can't just do something that popped up in your head a few seconds ago. The best way is to plan your activity ahead of time and mark it on your calendar. Put it somewhere you can easily see or put it in your agenda if you have one. Be sure, however, to stick to one rule - you're not just simply planning and jotting it down on the calendar – you are *committing* to it. You are not allowed to cancel unless there is an emergency. I love glancing at my calendar for the week and seeing my fun activity on my schedule – something to look forward to!

Now let's dive into the best part of this chapter - the long list of things that we moms can apply every week. Don't get nervous as these activities won't break the bank!

Take a Day Off from Cooking

Like professional chefs in a 5-star gourmet restaurant, moms too spend hours upon hours in the kitchen. It's safe to say that we try our best to cook every day to provide the best meals for our families. Cooking for our little monkeys might sound simple to other people, but truth be told, it can be extra stressful sometimes - especially when you have no idea what to cook for the day! Why not take one night off from working in the kitchen? Get on the phone and order takeout instead. You've been preparing all breakfasts, lunches, and dinners just about every day of the week, so nothing's wrong with ordering food to be delivered to your doorstep once a week if you're able. I'm pretty sure your kids wouldn't mind digging into a few slices of pepperoni pizza once in a while – needless to say, my kids love it! They eat something different at least once a week, and I get to rest, away from the kitchen. Of course, you can take them out as well. The important thing is to give yourself the night off from cooking...and cleaning!

Immerse Yourself in the Great Outdoors

Besides listening to music and meditating, surrounding yourself with nature can also help you release the unlimited stress lingering in your mind. So, get up early in the morning, grab a water bottle and a light snack and make your way to the nearest nature park around your neighborhood. Take advantage of the beautiful weather and check out a new trail. You can plug in your earphones and listen to your favorite music or just enjoy the sounds of nature - birds chirping and wind rustling through the trees. You'll be surprised at how fast you can get distracted from your problems by doing this.

Time in nature doesn't require you to be alone. You can bring your kids if you'd like and explore the outdoors together. It'll be good for them as well - at least they're doing something healthier than staring at their screens 24/7. Up for more of a challenge? Grab your hiking boots, lace up, and trek through a more grueling trail. You'll end up with a bucket of sweat, of course, but you can't deny the feeling of sweet satisfaction once you reach your destination.

Enroll in Free Online Courses

We're in the 21st century, and signing up for a course to learn something new is just a click away. The words "online course" might scare some people because who wants to sit for an hour listening to a lecture from instructors babbling about boring facts?! Don't let that fool you as there is a wide variety of fun online courses that you can explore these days - not the type where you'll be needing a notebook and a pen, entirely focused.

Go online and search for a course about your hobbies or interests. If you're not into learning foreign languages, don't force yourself to participate in a Chinese language course. If you love taking pictures of your food and posting it on your Instagram, you could find a free online course that teaches you how to take better photographs of your subject. You can learn all about angles, lighting, editing, and many other details about photography. Do you feel like painting but are unsure about a particular technique of blending colors? There are endless tutorials online and what's best is that many of them are free. You can simply go on YouTube, follow step-by-step painting tutorial videos by Bob Ross or many other instructors. So don't let the words "online course" scare you, as these courses can relieve stress and act as a self-care activity. Who knows, maybe as you're exploring these online courses, you might stumble upon a business idea for a home-based side-hustle!

Spend Time with Friends

We might not meet our friends as often as we did in our early adulthood. Having a family might mean more time at home with them, but that doesn't mean we can't have a girls' day out occasionally. If you enjoy wine, a lovely evening at a wine bar with a couple of close friends sounds perfect. But how about the children at home? Who's going to look after them? Well, before planning this, let your partner know of your plans and let him take the wheel. If you have a child who's old enough to be left at home alone with their younger siblings, then let the inmates run the asylum! Just make sure to set a few ground rules, so you don't return home looking as if a tornado had struck.

If wine is not for you, you can always opt to hit the spa with your girlfriends. You can book a manicure and pedicure session, get a traditional massage to ease your back pain or a facial, and enjoy the day. Another fantastic idea without spending too much money is to host a moms' appetizer and dessert night. Everyone can bring something either savory or sweet. Your kids can have a playdate with your friends' children while you have a catch-up session with your fellow moms. Nothing can clear a mind better than a few good laughs with your friends.

DATE NIGHT WITH YOUR PARTNER

Planning a date night with your significant other is not as easy as it seems, especially when you're surrounded by little clones created by you. If you don't have the budget to call in a babysitter for your children, you can try and ask your friendly neighbor or a close friend to watch the kids for an hour or two. When the boys were younger, we had a babysitting swap with our neighbors down the street. One week we would watch their kids while they went out, and next time, we would reciprocate. Babysitting can get expensive, so keeping costs down like this helps a bit. Unfortunately for my neighbors, they got the raw end of the deal. While we got to babysit their calm and angelic kids, they had to deal with our rambunctious boys!

Now that the kids are away and you have a couple of hours to enjoy with your other half, go ahead and have fun like when you went out on your first date! It might be as simple as watching a rom-com on the flatscreen, or you could go the extra mile and check out that new restaurant in town. You don't always get to do this without having the little ones calling for you every second, so enjoy it to the fullest!

DATE NIGHT WITH YOURSELF

When I needed a few hours to myself to unwind at the end of the week, I used to send the boys to their grandparents' house. My sons were more than happy to spend time with them. Whether you're a single mom like me or just want some time off alone, the solitude can be refreshing.

If you have an eye for art, grab your car keys and drive to an art museum in your area. Walk around from one section to the next, admire the masterpieces, and enjoy the peaceful environment.

You can also unleash your inner shopaholic self by going to garage sales or thrift stores. This way, you won't be spending hundreds of dollars and feeling guilty afterward. Garage sales and thrift stores usually have unique trinkets and treasures reasonably priced, so don't hold yourself back and feel free to browse through the items that catch your eye.

SLEEP IN

Waking up early in the morning every day can be dreadful at times, so it's not wrong for you to sleep in every once in a while. Instead of waking up at 6 a.m., set the alarm clock to 8 a.m. or don't set the alarm at all. Tell your kids not to disturb your beauty sleep unless it's an emergency. Remind them that finding a misplaced toy is not considered 'extremely important,' so don't let them wake you up because of that.

Your body needs rest, too - you can't risk yourself being sleep-deprived and slowly falling into the dark hole of fatigue and exhaustion. So, moms, start planning your weekly self-care routine now. Applying these weekly routines can massively contribute to your mental health. You'll get to return to your daily tasks as a mom the following week with a fresh mind and a recharged body.

Other than the ideas listed above, here are more activities that you can plan and look forward to:

- declutter a small part of your house
- try out a new recipe you just discovered
- set a picnic by the beach (alone or with your kids)
- visit the library or a bookstore and discover a new book or genre
- sit in a coffee shop doing nothing but sipping a hot latte
- watch a few funny videos on YouTube
- take a long, warm shower with your go-to karaoke song playing in the background
- reorganize or redecorate a space in your house
- try out a new hobby
- clear out your wardrobe, set the things you no

longer need aside, and donate them to those in need

- visit a nursery and get yourself a new houseplant
- join a pottery class
- treat yourself to your favorite food and eat it by the beach or somewhere serene
- pick up a new musical instrument and enroll in a class
- bake colorful macarons and share them with your friends and neighbors
- buy a sushi-making kit and learn how to make sushi rolls
- host a game night for family and friends
- take the kids to an arcade and join them

FIVE

EVERY NOW AND THEN

I'm not sure about you, but I would do anything to avoid burnout, as that was one of the worst experiences I have had since becoming a mom. It felt like I was at my lowest during that unfortunate time, as if a strong, sturdy brick wall around me had utterly collapsed, leaving me feeling more vulnerable than ever. The signs of exhaustion were written all over my face. I thought to myself, a power nap was all I needed, but little did I know back then that it'll keep on repeatedly happening unless I did something to stop it.

After a few consultations with medical professionals and some time spent researching how to eliminate burnout, I concluded that I seriously needed to reorganize my schedule. I started to change my morning routine by inserting a few short activities that could boost my mind every day. After convincing myself that self-care is not a selfish act, I created and planned my weekly activity and actually *did* it. When I planned to go explore a new walking trail on Saturday morning, I committed to what I intended. It takes time - I'm not even going to lie about it - but I gradually felt better when sticking to these routines.

I began, however, to experience significant positive changes when I stepped up the game a little bit. Every once in a while, I would go on a short getaway and take a couple of days off from piloting the family. According to my therapist, going on trips will allow the kids to miss you, and it can be a good break for them, too. My favorite part of doing this is when I return home and get smothered with piles of affection and tight hugs from them! Of course, this might be a more elaborate self-care activity. You'll need a higher budget, so make sure to save accordingly. I squirrel away a bit of my budget each month towards these getaways, so it doesn't make a crazy dent in my finances. You can get creative and use any reward points you may have with your credit cards as well. But don't worry, there are many other things you can do other than going on a vacation.

Weekend Getaway with Friends or Spouse

Ready your bags and hit the road! After settling your children first, of course. You can either do this with your spouse or your closest friends. Choose a suitable destination - preferably somewhere you won't have to fight traffic to get there. I like to start my time leaving Friday morning and returning Sunday evening. Of course, a simple overnighter would be fine as well. This time away can be considered a short vacation, so make the most of it like you would whenever you were on a holiday way back before you had kids.

Google unique eateries serving inventive food. Make a list of the restaurants you want to visit and seize the day. I often plan my trips around food! Jump from one place to another, satisfy your cravings, and let yourself be free for a while. Take a trip to a local vineyard for some wine tasting or perhaps explore a wine cave. Anything that comes to mind - as long as it's beneficial and relaxing for you - just do it. You don't get this chance to have a blast every week!

Nature Retreat

One of the best ways to release stress and refresh your mind is to have a retreat away from the bustling concrete jungle. Instead of listening to the sounds of cars honking and noisy crowds everywhere, go on the Airbnb app and book a place surrounded by nature where the only things you wake up to are calming sounds of birds chirping and streams flowing down the cascades. Fill up your itinerary with outdoor activities, so you get revitalized with fresh air in your system. Go on a trail to a waterfall or hike up a mountain and be greeted by a spectacular view of your surroundings.

While immersing yourself in the quiet environment, you can also spend the day doing things you love - from painting to meditating, writing, and even sleeping - you can do anything since it's *your* retreat. This is the perfect time for you to unwind and relax completely. So, don't let anyone stop you. You deserve this, mama!

Catch a Movie

Instead of watching shows on your flatscreen like any other day, take advantage of this time off and head to the theater. Choose a newly-released Hollywood movie you've been dying to see, walk up to the concession stand, and get yourself a bucket of sweet caramel popcorn or some nachos to enjoy during the movie.

Volunteering

Believe it or not, volunteering, too, can count as self-care, and what's even better is that you won't even need to spend a massive amount of money on it.

I'm sure there are a lot of volunteer opportunities you can find in your neighborhood. If you're a wildlife enthusiast, sign up to volunteer at the zoo. If you love cooking, you can join a non-profit organization that hosts hunger relief programs. Aside from gaining a new experience, regularly volunteering also plays a part in improving your mental health - it helps you reduce stress and depression. It can even help people to overcome the loss of a loved one.

You can try and do these activities at least once every few months. Remember, moms, save your budgets accordingly! You might want to plan something more special than usual every once in a while to have something exciting to look forward to. However, keep in mind that how you will be spending your time away is entirely up to you. If you can't seem to go for a short getaway due to your financial situation, don't force yourself - it'll only lead to more stress. Instead, look for other alternatives that won't hurt your bank account.

Here are some other ideas that you can consider while you're planning your getaway:

- go on an overnight near an aquarium
- rent an RV and live the van life for a weekend
- take a train trip to a nearby city
- glamp on the beach
- reserve a cabin in the mountains
- send the kids to their grandparents and live it up
  like a tourist in your town

SIX

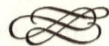

DON'T GO IT ALONE

ou are not alone, and you will never be!

Moms, please take these words and lock them in your memory. There are close to eight billion people globally, so it is nearly impossible for you to be alone. Remember that there is always someone willing to help you go through the rough patches in your life. If you've tried everything within your power to bring yourself back up, but you can't seem to see any positive changes, then it's time to seek help from someone other than yourself. We, moms, are no different than other human beings - we too can get exhausted, stressed out, anxious, pressured, and everything in between. So, there's nothing wrong with us reaching out seeking help. Doing this doesn't mean that we are weak, so swallow your pride and don't be afraid to ask for help.

If you ever find yourself extremely overwhelmed, the first person that you should turn to is, of course, your spouse. At certain times, all we need is just someone to talk to. So, don't be afraid to let it all out. Tell your partner how you are feeling and what things occupy your mind the most. Try to come up with a solution together. People want to help you most of the time, but they just don't know how unless you communicate with them. At this moment, it's best to avoid beating around the bush so that both of you will be on the same page.

Besides your spouse, you can also turn to friends or your other family members - especially the grandparents to your children. If you desperately need a short escape or alone time away from the daily chores, don't feel guilty to request help from the grandparents or other close family members. Not only will you be granted some alone time, but doing this will also allow your children to bond with their grandparents – it's a win/win!

I've also found church groups within my community to be a great resource to meet other moms to lean on for support. If anyone should understand the challenges you're going through, it's a fellow mama.

And when you need it, you can always seek help from professional therapists if you feel your mental state declining and if it appears to be almost impossible for you to snap out of it. People often get spooked whenever it is suggested to meet with a therapist because, for some, seeing a psychologist is equivalent to suffering from a mental illness. But it's time to remove that misconception as therapy is for everyone. You don't have to suffer from a severe mental illness to make an appointment. Therapists are also certified professionals, so they can provide you with great solutions and options to explore. Anyone who feels consumed by stress and intense emotions should book a session. Talking to a therapist offers you a safe, non-judgmental place where you can talk about the experiences and worries wreaking havoc in your mind.

See, mama? You're not alone in this! Keeping everything to yourself will only make it worse. People around you, perhaps your friendly neighbors next door or your church community, are more than happy to assist you. They are likely willing to lend a hand but won't know you need help until you reach out.

SPECIAL REQUEST

PAY IT FORWARD AND HELP OTHER WORN-OUT MOMS FIND THIS BOOK!

Have you found some key strategies to reclaiming your sanity? Would you like to help other moms do the same?

I hope you've enjoyed *Self-Care Strategies for 24/7 Moms* so far. Before we wrap it up with my final words, I would be incredibly thankful if you would leave a brief review or rating for this book wherever you purchased it – even if it's just a few short sentences.

You never know who you might be helping by leaving your review. Your words just might encourage a weary mom to make the necessary changes her family needs for a better home life!

Thank you!

FINAL WORDS

~

Parenthood is obviously not as easy as it sounds. Being a mom comes in a package of overwhelming duties and continuous challenges. Your journey began as soon as those two lines appeared on that pregnancy test. You may encounter various barriers that might bring you down, but as long as you can find the time to put yourself first, the chances of you getting thrown into the pit of exhaustion and burnout will be minimized.

Introducing self-care into your daily life might sound simple, but you could easily give up if you're not following the proper steps. As I said before, you have to begin with baby steps as you make self-care a part of your new normal. So, be patient, start with simple morning routines, and fill up your precious time with small activities that can put a smile on your face. Remember that self-care is personal, and certain practices that work for others might not necessarily work for you. It's entirely up to you to organize your schedule and choose self-care ideas that will suit you best.

Now that you have taken steps to apply self-care into your life as a loving mother, there's no going back! Don't let a single soul stop you from taking care of yourself. Of utmost importance, don't feel guilty. Keep telling yourself that self-care is not a selfish act and you *need* it to care for your family. If you can't take proper care of yourself, you can't expect to provide complete care to your children - it all starts with *you*.

So, go, mama! Make some time for yourself, and don't allow an ounce of guilt stop you. You don't want to wake up in the morning noticing a new wrinkle on your face each day and fighting with your mood swings until the sun sets. No one says that setting a foot into motherhood means we must stop living our life to the fullest. Who says we must sacrifice our hobbies to take good care of our family? That's right, no one! So, continue doing whatever you love - hike up a hill, try out new recipes, knit a blanket, paint that scenery, visit museums, and everything in between. As long as it's beneficial for you, then why not? After all, a happy mother makes a home brighter.

I truly hope you can make use of the tips included in this book and successfully achieve the perfect balance between rest and responsibility while continuing to provide loving care for your family!

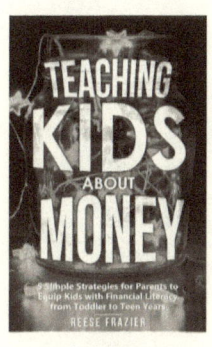

Finance Crash Course for College Students and Young Adults. How to Manage Money, Save Money Fast, Pay off Debt, and Invest in the Stock Market

REFERENCES

Eating Well for Mental Health. (n.d.). Sutter Health. https://www.sutterhealth.org/health/nutrition/eating-well-for-mental-health

Hjalmarsdottir, F. (2018, October 14). *17 Science-Based Benefits of Omega-3 Fatty Acids*. Healthline. https://www.healthline.com/nutrition/17-health-benefits-of-omega-3

Locricchio, S. (2018, January 22). *The Dangers of Neglecting Self-Care*. Wellness Warriors Revolution. https://wellnesswarriorsrevolution.com/dangers-neglecting-self-care/

McDermott, A. (2019, March 7). *Try this: 18 Essential Oils for Anxiety*. Healthline. https://www.healthline.

com/health/anxiety/essential-oils-for-anxiety#chamomile

Nazish, N. (2019, March 8). *Five Totally Doable Self-Care Tips for Busy Moms*. Forbes. https://www.forbes.com/sites/nomanazish/2019/03/08/five-totally-doable-self-care-tips-for-busy-moms/?sh=9a9d9db1d753

Sean, J. (n.d.). *10 Surprising Benefits of Morning Exercises (backed by science)*. Daily Healthy Body. https://www.dailyhealthybody.com/fitness/morning-exercise-benefits/

Steiss, T. (n.d.). *The Surprising Mandala Coloring Benefits for Adults*. Happiness.Com. https://www.happiness.com/magazine/art-culture-leisure/mandala-coloring-benefits/

ABOUT THE AUTHOR

~

Based in Southern California, Reese Frazier is a mom of three boys who loves God/family/travel/wine/food/dogs naps (ideal weekends include a combination of these). She has managed to keep her sanity while single-parenting her sons (born within four years of each other). Reese is passionate about self-care and firmly believes it is critical to the family's well-being as a whole.